Resistance band Workout:

The ultimate solution to getting stronger, faster and healthier

Roger Hutchinson

Table of contents

Chapter 1

What you should know about resistance bands

Workout resistance bands have been a fixture of exercise programs for both muscled-up gym veterans and fitness training beginners. The reason? They're simple to use, incredibly adaptable, and tremendously effective.

No matter what your fitness level, resistance bands are a terrific piece of equipment to utilize.

So don't let the simplicity of resistance bands mislead you. There's a perfect manner to utilize the bands in order to receive their muscle-building advantage. Let's go over some pointers and exercises

What is resistance band training?

With resistance band training, you substitute cumbersome workout equipment with rubber resistance bands that you stretch. The effort it requires to stretch the bands develops your muscles exactly like using free weights or machines.

Resistance bands make working out convenient and super-effective. They exert a steady pressure on your muscles and you may carry them discreetly to burst out some rapid workout wherever you are when you find the time.

Yet finding the proper resistance band for the task might be tricky. Navigating the many designs and resistance levels is crucial to obtaining the greatest exercise possible, therefore it's important to know and appreciate not just how various resistance band models are distinct but also how you can use them in your daily regimen to push your muscles to their limits.

Read on to find out all you need to know about the five kinds of resistance bands, which one you should pick based on your fitness objectives, and how you can integrate them into your exercise safely and successfully.

DO RESISTANCE BANDS WORK?

Resistance bands are particularly effective in opposing muscular action so that fibers have to exert themselves, causing the damage that is so necessary for strength gains and muscle development via hypertrophy.

We like to imagine bodybuilders working out with massive weight plates on each end of barbells or lifting huge tires to become chiseled and ripped. While they're modest, resistance bands may assist create comparable outcomes.

Of all, even the toughest resistance band doesn't give the same challenge as very heavy weights do. If you're already an accomplished lifter, you'll undoubtedly need to add typical strength training routines to your daily workout program. For most individuals, resistance bands will be adequate to accomplish their exercise objectives.

It's also feasible to add resistance bands in many strength training activities. For example, you might put a resistance band around each end of a barbell and below the bench to make bench presses more difficult during the whole exercise.

HOW DO RESISTANCE BANDS WORK?

Manufacturers often employ synthetic rubber, latex, or comparable material to manufacture their resistance bands. Several additionally weave in elastic fabric to make their latex bands more comfortable and less prone to slide and roll.

The suppleness of the band is important to how it operates. You may either wrap the band around two portions of your body or fasten it to an anchor point such that movement away from one end of the band causes strain. This tension generates resistance against your muscles, pushing them to work harder to execute a specific activity.

When you expand the range of motion of an exercise, the resistance from the band rises. The practical implication of this linear rise in resistance is that you may continuously enhance the performance of your muscles in an immensely useful manner. There's no better way to develop your range of motion than to consistently practice going through that range of motion under the continuous pressure a resistance band offers.

5 TYPES OF RESISTANCE BANDS

Generally speaking, resistance bands fall into one of the following five groups. Many companies design unique variations on these five or use proprietary materials to make their product stand out against the competition, but if you're looking for the right kind of resistance band to suit your workout routine and fitness goals, understanding these 5 types is a good place to start.

1. LOOP BANDS

Perhaps the most popular tool for resistance band exercises, the loop band is basic in manufacturing and enticing in its adaptability. They're really simply giant rubber bands that you can fasten to an anchor point, wrap around your arms and legs, or even attach to free weights to make regular strength training routines tougher.

Resistance loops are helpful for bodyweight activities like push-ups because you can wrap them over your shoulders to provide more challenges without having to add extra weight. In the case of the push-up, adding weight any other way is fairly impossible.

Loop bands are the simplest to get into position for an activity. If you need to establish an anchor point, you may simply fold them in half around a vertical or horizontal bar and draw one end through to form a knot. With a big enough loop band, you may connect dumbbells and other weights to an anchor point or step on the other end of the band to produce greater stress.

2. MINI BANDS

These resistance bands appear like loop bands only they're a little broader and often considerably smaller. You wouldn't use them to build up anchor points or add tension to weight training exercises as you would with loop bands, however. Rather, you would wrap them around your legs for most workouts or your wrists for a few others.

You may hear folks nickname them booty bands since they're typically utilized for lower-body workouts that will give you amazing glutes. Small bands are wrapped around the legs above the knees or around the ankles to accomplish this advantage.

Generally speaking, these exercise bands are less beneficial for targeting muscle groups in the upper body since they aren't large enough to wrap over your shoulders. But, you may attach small bands over both wrists to add tension to bodyweight lat pulldowns. This is very beneficial when you can't establish a door anchor or tie a longer band to a high anchor point as you need to execute band pulldowns.

Another alternative is to wrap the tiny band around one arm by bending your elbow and moving the band up until it's near your wrist and armpit at either end. This will increase strain on bicep curls. You might also wrap micro bands around a bar to establish an anchor point for triceps curls, but their small size makes them less handy for this purpose than a big loop band would be.

3. TUBE BANDS

Tube resistance bands are created with grips on one end and a tiny loop on the other for simple connection at anchor points. The elastic bands are not as broad and are more circular, more like ropes than flatter loop bands and tiny bands.

Rather than looping them around both legs as you would with loop resistance bands, you would use tube bands to apply tension to workouts that require you to move a body component away from a fixed external point. For example, a tube resistance band might be more useful for lower body activities like the standing lateral leg raise.

You may also use a tube resistance band to work and exercise the muscular groups in your upper body. Putting up door anchors is quick and straightforward, and it's much easier to retain a grasp utilizing the grips on tube resistance bands.

Tube bands with grips make workouts like the banded chest press simple to complete with the appropriate technique.

One specific sort of tube band is called the Figure 8 Band. It's just two loops with a bridge in the center - envision a loop band with a constrictor piece in the middle that produces two loops. There are grips on the outside of each loop, making them excellent for pull-apart exercises with the loops held by your hands or as ankle straps over your feet.

4. THERAPY BANDS

Individuals with an injury history, receiving physical therapy, or in need of additional light-impact resistance band training commonly utilize therapeutic bands, which are similar to loop bands but aren't attached at the ends. While they're tougher to grasp than loop or tube bands when used for less strenuous workouts therapeutic bands are gentler on the joints and hands.

The elderly and persons visiting physical therapists are likely to utilize these bands, but many others also like therapeutic bands for their warm-ups and cool-down exercises after their primary regimen is over. Utilizing the light-resistance therapeutic band for the warm-up and higher-tension versions for the main program helps minimize persistent stiffness or soreness and also helps exhaust some of the slow-twitch muscles that are most resistant to exhaustion.

Therapy bands may be connected together to replicate the advantages of normal loop bands, however, all that tying and untying, as well as the danger of tying a knot you can't untie, might make them a less-than-ideal solution for some.

5. PULL-UP BANDS

Although most of the other bands on this list are used for various sorts of workouts, pull-up bands are specially constructed to support users' body weights during pull-ups and chin-ups. Many individuals utilize them to attain that elusive first pull-up or conquer plateaus in their pull-up count. They're simply enormous, heavy-duty loop bands that can sustain the majority of a person's body weight.

Resistance bands exert greater pressure the more they're stretched, which offers a weird challenge for folks who use pull-up bands as part of their routine. The band is designed to be used by connecting it to the horizontal pull-up bar and then stepping onto it with one or both feet - the resistance band is what supports the body weight of the user.

Yet it also implies that the band offers the greatest support for the user while they're in the lowest position, i.e. the simplest phase of the exercise. When you push your body toward the pull-up bar, the band gives less aid.

Nonetheless, they are beneficial for helping you conserve some strength so you can utilize them to perform a pull-up. It's sort of like batting with a doughnut in that you can develop the strength to assist you to go through more bandless pull-ups.

Resistance bands make working out convenient and super-effective. They exert a steady pressure on your muscles and you may carry them discretely to burst out some rapid workout wherever you are when you find the time.

Yet finding the proper resistance band for the task might be tricky. Navigating the many designs and resistance levels is crucial to obtaining the greatest exercise possible, therefore it's important to know and appreciate not just how various resistance band models are distinct but also how you can use them in your daily regimen to push your muscles to their limits.

Read on to find out all you need to know about the five kinds of resistance bands, which one you should pick based on your fitness objectives, and how you can integrate them into your exercise safely and successfully.

THE BEST RESISTANCE BAND FOR A TOUGH WORKOUT

So, with all these various kinds of resistance bands, which one is the greatest for generating toned muscles and functional strength?

If you're seeking adaptability, loop bands are the ideal option. Tube bands may include handles that make them easier to grasp, but regular loop bands will assist improve grip strength and ultimately will become easy enough to hold onto. You may also knot loop bands to construct anchor points as quickly as you might link the loop end of a tube band to an anchor.

Loop bands allow you to increase tension to more sorts of workouts. For instance, you might use them around your legs or wrap them over your arms. They can be grabbed for pull-apart or linked to an anchor point for pulldowns, or you could even wrap them around barbells and free weights to add some resistance training to your strength training regimen.

There are a few circumstances when you could select one of the other kinds of resistance bands. You surely need a pull-up band to execute band-assisted pull-ups. You also may want tiny microbands if you're practicing isometrics. Pilates and therapeutic bands are a traditional combo.

In most cases, loop bands do the work, which is why they're the greatest all-around sort of resistance band. But the others may come in helpful occasionally as well, which is why it's better to invest in a resistance band set that offers a range of kinds. They're affordable, particularly compared to heavy-duty strength training equipment, so purchasing an entire set shouldn't put you back too much.

HOW TO CHOOSE THE RIGHT LEVEL OF RESISTANCE

Navigating the numerous degrees of resistance offered on these bands isn't as straightforward as it seems. Some of the guidelines are obvious - mild resistance when you first start and steadily increased degrees of resistance as you grow stronger, for example.

You may also utilize varied degrees of resistance within one training regimen to drive certain muscle areas into exhaustion.

Using a less resistant band for bicep curls to totally exhaust your biceps following a full-body exercise with high-level resistance bands can assist you to promote hypertrophy.

Overdoing it on the resistance band might undermine some of the best benefits of utilizing resistance bands in the first place. The bands frequently help users complete workouts with far better form than they would normally, especially when they're learning new techniques.

But choose a band that offers you more resistance than you need and it might actively inhibit you from executing exercises with the appropriate form.

That's another solid reason why you should invest in a set of several sorts of resistance bands.

Having several styles and strengths with you means you won't cheat yourself out of a workout - you can always switch to a different style or vary the amount of resistance to suit your demands at a particular time.

Most manufacturers color-mark their resistance bands so that you know what amount of resistance you have.

It's handy for quickly picking the band you need, so as long as you select a set that contains all the colors you need, you'll be prepared for exercises of various complexity and just much any banded activity you can think to put in.

The most crucial thing in picking the proper amount of resistance is to try them out and listen to your body as you begin using your new exercise equipment. If your muscles are fatiguing too rapidly or you aren't getting the results you desire, reassess the bands you're using.

STARTING OUT WITH RESISTANCE BANDS

If you're still in the initial stages of introducing resistance bands into your exercises, tube bands with handles can be the ideal option until you get the hang of all the routines and build up enough grip strength to utilize loop bands. For certain workouts, you may never want to convert from the tube band to a loop band or another kind.

Incorporating resistance bands into bodyweight exercise programs is a little less challenging than doing the same with strength training exercises.

If the ease of bands is what appeals to you most, you may want to look into substituting the equipment-dependent routines with their resistance band equivalents so that you can get the same fantastic workout without having to invest in a home gym with loads of gear and equipment.

Start putting resistance band exercises into your workouts by integrating them into your warm-up regimen. This will also help you gain strength for more challenging exercises and nail the technique so you can give your muscles the greatest and most focused workout possible.

Knowing how to use resistance bands correctly is also vital for preventing things like slapbacks, which hurt rather intensely and might cause injuries that will pull you out of your exercise program for weeks or more if they're serious enough.

CONCLUSION

Resistance bands usage is an intense method to make your exercise tougher and push your muscles to their limits. The strain they create on your muscles not only helps them work harder but also allows you to target them from various angles that aren't achievable with weights alone.

The bands come in numerous forms and degrees of resistance so you may adapt your regimen to reach your fitness objectives. Progressive overload and other approaches for hypertrophy are very much doable with resistance bands alone, or you may couple them with weights to make strength training routines more of a challenge.

Loop bands are by far the greatest type because of their adaptability, although the other forms come in helpful in specific circumstances.

Invest in a set of resistance bands that has different types and strengths and you'll be able to reach your strength gains and fitness objectives in no time.

Advantages of resistance bands

Resistance bands were developed as a technique for nursing home patients to gain strength. Gradually, they became much more widespread as people realized the advantages of exercising with these gigantic rubber bands.

Benefits of resistance bands include:

Adaptability. You may alter exercises on the fly by adjusting motions to test your muscles in various ways. And workout bands enable you to raise or reduce resistance simply by shortening or extending the band.

Portability. Resistance bands may simply fit in a travel carry bag to enable you to work out anywhere you may wonder. As for conventional weights ... well, you're not getting that through a TSA screening.

Cost. A solid set of resistance bands costs significantly less than comparable strength-training equipment.

Are resistance bands useful for weight loss?

Exercising with resistance bands doesn't only develop muscle. It may also help melt away fat.

Research published in 2022 reveals that resistance band training decreases body fat in those who are overweight better than other kinds of training, including free weights and bodyweight activities. The evaluation looked at 18 studies including 669 people.

How to start using resistance bands

Resistance bands vary from basic, flat treatment bands to flat loop bands and elastic tubing with replaceable handles that make them more user-friendly.

Select a set of bands with varied resistances, or tension levels. Bands generally are color-coded, with increased tension given as the band colors go darker. (Greater tension is the equivalent of more weight, to put it in lifting words.)

The more strength that's necessary for an activity, the greater the resistance you'll need from the band. (As an example, you'll need more tension for a chest press than a bicep curl, notes Travers.)

Additionally, evaluate the sorts of accessories that come with the bands, such as door attachments or ankle cuffs, and match them with the types of activity you want to undertake.

Additional tips include:

Wear shoes anytime you use resistance bands to prevent sliding.

When you link a band to a door, give it a solid pull before you work out to be sure it's secure.

Periodically examine bands for indications of wear and tear. If they've been exposed to a lot of light or cold, they may shatter.

Emphasis on technique

Don't add too much resistance for an exerciser or you won't have a smooth range of motion. You'll profit more by employing excellent form with lesser resistance than by attempting to boost the tension level.

"With any sort of exercise, you have to maintain appropriate form and posture, just as you would if you were using an exercise machine. And the reps and resistance may fluctuate dependent on the person. Simply take your muscles to tiredness to get the most out of a session."

As you gain more familiarity with moves, it's good to push yourself by increasing the tension on the resistance bands. Just make sure your form doesn't break down as you move up a level.

A word of caution, too: Don't overstretch bands to attempt to create resistance. It may cause a band to shatter and lead to possible injury.

Chapter 2

Things to note as a beginner aiming for fitness

If you've wanted to start strength training, but didn't know where to begin, utilizing resistance bands is a good way to start.

How Long and How Frequently Should You Perform Resistance Band Training?

When starting resistance band workouts, you'll want to aim for two strength-based training sessions every week that are about 30 minutes each, according to the International Sports Science Association (ISSA)–certified personal trainer Mike Matthews, author of Muscle for Life: Get Lean, Strong, and Healthy at Any Age! "You can make a lot of progress on two exercises per week [on nonconsecutive days], especially if your objective is to move from unfit to fit," he adds.

This applies to persons who are newcomers to exercise, as well as those who are already routinely working out, but new to resistance band training. The difference (we'll get to this later) is the intensity of your workout.

This level of strength training coincides with guidelines from the U.S. Department of Health and Human Services that urge individuals to practice strength exercises two or more days per week that concentrate on all major muscle groups.

(They include legs, back, belly, chest, shoulders, and arms.)

If you're already doing cardio, you can squeeze in a resistance band exercise on "off" cardio days. Another alternative is to complete both exercises in one day, doing exercise band training first, followed by cardio. Preferably you want to adhere to this schedule so your muscles aren't too burned out from the cardio to undertake the strength training.

If you're currently performing other strength exercises, you may add resistance band workouts into your weekly program or swap an existing strength session with one utilizing bands.

Items You Need for Resistance Band Workouts

The equipment and gear required for a resistance band exercise are relatively simple.

Resistance Bands: This is the obvious one, right? It's better if you have a few resistance bands that vary in the amount of resistance (or stretchiness) (or stretchiness). There are numerous kinds available, from looped to ribbons and those with handles. Select the one that is most comfortable and easiest to use. (Considering the workouts you could be utilizing the bands for will help you select.)

Clothes: You Can Move and Sweat In Gear up with breathable, comfortable gear that you can move about in, and won't feel too heavy when your body begins to heat up.

And these items of gear and equipment are optional but may make some workouts simpler to accomplish

Sneakers: Most resistance band workouts may be done barefoot. But if you are on a surface where you could slide or you feel more comfortable, confident, and balanced in shoes, try lacing up.

Yoga Mat: For on-the-ground workouts, it may assist avoid sliding and offer some cushioning if you're on a hard floor.

Safety Tips for Resistance Band Workouts

In general, resistance bands are very safe to use, especially when you start out with a band that has a low resistance.

The benefits outweigh the risks, as long as you start easy and ramp up slowly. Whether you are recovering from an accident, or surgery, or have a chronic health condition, it's always a good idea to consult with your doctor before beginning a new fitness routine.

Progressing gradually in resistance, intensity, and amount of exercises is the safest method. "If you've never used a resistance band before and you immediately start cranking out tons of reps on a heavy resistance, you could definitely be at an increased risk for developing tendinitis, bursitis, or another overuse injury," says Brendan Martin, PT, DPT, a physical therapist with Finish Line Physical Therapy in New York City.

Yet, there's a simple solution: If a technique seems too intense right from the start with a band, don't utilize it. Add a band after you're able to securely complete the motion. If the activity involves completing squats with a looped resistance band put around the thighs, but you're unable to finish one repetition (rep) with the band, execute the set without the band. After the set begins to seem less tough, consider adding the band.

Another safety consideration is: Prevent harm from inappropriate usage of the band. Certain routines may need you to tie a resistance band to an anchor point (such as a tree outdoors or a beam in your house or gym) (like a tree outside or a beam in your home or gym). When that's the case, make sure the anchor point is sturdy. Tying it to a kitchen table or chair, for instance, implies that you'll pull that piece of furniture toward you.

Additionally, pay attention to the health of the bands themselves. Resistant bands do wear out. As they near the end of their existence, they frequently snap and start flying. Always check to make sure your band isn't beginning to rip.

The consequence of a projectile band is that there's a genuine danger one may snap back and strike you in the face. If a band snaps into your eye it might cause harm, for instance, causing retinal detachment, which is a medical emergency.

Before using it, make sure that you have a strong grasp of the band. And if you do strike your eye, it's a good idea to consult an ophthalmologist if you have eye discomfort, issues with vision, seeing flashes of light or floaters, or problems with eye movement.

How to Warm Up for Resistance Band Workouts

Before your workout, warm up your body with a quick, fast walk. You might also attempt active stretches, such as a few squats, lunges, and arm circles. "These let your body know it will be working out," he explains. The idea is to get your muscles feeling loosened up before you start stressing them more strongly with particular workouts.

In addition, it's essential to begin each session with a few minutes of balancing training, says Joyner. This could entail standing next to a table (holding onto it if required) and elevating one knee hip-height and holding it, standing tall. You may alternatively stand in a wide stance and gently move to one side, elevating the opposing foot.

Performing balance training is beneficial in improving daily function, as well as helping you maintain safe movement patterns in resistance exercise. Balancing exercise teaches your neuromuscular system to remain stable on your feet during each action, which eventually enhances the safety of the activity.

Chapter 3

Resistance band workouts for chest

The chest muscles might be regarded as a distinguishing feature of strong anatomy. They are engaged in acts such as squeezing a set of loppers to cut a tree limb and pushing a door open. These are also the key muscles addressed when arguing upper body strength.

For bodybuilders and those interested in general physical aesthetics, the chest muscles are the defining component of muscle mass. Powerlifters depend on them for the bench press to score the biggest lift.

Yet these muscles are also highly essential from a functional aspect since they assist the movement of the arms.

A number of studies assessing perceived attractiveness indicated that a low waist-to-chest ratio was considered the most appealing physical trait in guys. This is when a person has a smaller waist and a larger chest.

Yet gender-specific beauty standards aside, everyone may benefit from strengthening the chest muscles – whether your objective is to have sculpted pecs or just to be able to play Twister with your kids on the living room floor.

What are the muscles of the chest?

There are three basic muscles that make up the chest:

pectoralis major
pectoralis minor
serratus anterior

A lesser-known muscle in the chest is called the subclavius. It is a tiny auxiliary muscle mostly engaged in respiration (breathing)

The pectoralis major is a remarkable muscle because it has two heads — the clavicular head and the sternocostal head. They are antagonistic to one another, which means that while one contracts, the other relaxes.

The clavicular head flexes the humerus, or upper arm bone, by elevating your arm in front of you. It also adducts the humerus — which means it pushes the arm inward toward the body's midline — and aids with the internal rotation of the same bone.

The sternocostal head, on the other hand, draws the arm down from a forward or flexed posture. It's also engaged in motions such as horizontal adduction (as if you were a bear-hugging someone) and internal rotation of the humerus.

The pectoralis minor's role is to support the shoulder blade by drawing it forward and down against the rib cage – a movement known as the protraction of the shoulder blade. It also improves shoulder stability and breathing.

The serratus anterior has a sawlike genesis on the outer front of the first through eighth ribs and finishes on the medial edge of the shoulder blade (closest to the spine) (closest to the spine). It drags the shoulder blade over the ribs to avoid scapular winging, giving stability to the shoulder during pushing actions.

Suggestions for defined chest muscles

"Muscle definition" is a hard phrase. You may question yourself, "What does it truly mean?"

Obviously, muscles have to expand in size to be able to perceive their form. This is termed hypertrophy, and it includes gradually straining the muscles beyond their resting condition to generate development.

It happens when the quantity of protein consumed to grow muscle surpasses the amount of protein breakdown that occurs.

But, you also need to reduce body fat to be able to show muscle definition. For persons with breasts, it will likely be difficult to discern much muscle definition in the chest.

Yet, if the muscular definition is your aim, you'll need to strengthen the chest muscles for hypertrophy but also reduce calories to show your muscles better. This would likely require boosting calorie burn via aerobic activity and regulating your diet

Let's begin

Be ready to say goodbye to free weights and hello to resistance bands... or at least to spice things up a bit. Variety is the spice of life, after all.

One study shows that resistance training using elastic bands may give equal strength improvements as exercising with dumbbells or weight machines. Here's how you get the greatest chest workout out of your resistance bands.

1. Banded floor press

No huge weights are required here. This floor press isolates your chest and triceps while reducing stress on your shoulders.

Try it:

Sit on the floor with knees pointing up and feet flat on the floor.
With one handle (or one end of the band) in each hand, put the resistance band across your back, beneath your shoulders.
Lay down on your back.
With palms towards the ceiling, push up until your arms are straight.

Slowly return your arms to the floor.
Try 10–12 repetitions.

Tips:

Keep your wrists straight to prevent injury.
Bring your hands closer together at the top
of the action.

2. Resistance band fly

Who doesn't appreciate a little tweak on a
classic? This exercise isolates your pectorals
for a super-focused workout.

Try it:

Locate something solid to wrap your
resistance band around, such as a pole or a
fence post.
Hold the handles or the ends of the band,
facing away from the pole.

Widen your stance. Hold arms out to the sides at chest level.
Maintaining a small bend in your elbows, bring your arms out in front of you.
Return your arms to the wide posture over a 3-second count.
Try 8–12 repetitions.

Tip: Keep your elbows underneath your shoulders.

3. Resistance band push-up

It's like a push-up but tougher. This exercise targets your chest and triceps to enhance upper-body strength.

Try it:

Put the resistance band around your back, beneath your shoulders.
Get into a plank stance.

Holding the plank posture, lower your body until it's barely over the floor.
Push back up. (You should feel the tightness of the resistance band at the height of the movement.)
Try 8–12 repetitions.

Tips:

If you're feeling bold, you can add a knee tuck for an added core exercise.
You can add a side knee tuck, too, but it's not for the faint of heart.

4. Straight-arm pulldown

Strong back and shoulder muscles assist support your chest during pressing exercises.

This exercise targets your latissimus dorsi (aka lats) and serratus anterior muscles and assists with scapular (shoulder) stability.

Try it:

Fasten the midpoint of the resistance band someplace a bit higher than your head. (Anything sturdy, like a door, will work — just make sure the door remains closed.)
Hold the ends of the band and take a few steps back, keeping your feet hip-width apart.
Lean your torso forward and preserve a small bend in your knees. Put your arms at a 45-degree angle in line with your ears.
With arms straight, bring the band down to your thighs and compress your lats.
Pause at the bottom, then gently release.
Try 10–12 repetitions.

Tips:

Try a resistance band door anchor. If you'll be performing this maneuver a lot, it's well worth the minor expense.

Lift your shoulders slightly down and back and try not to let them roll forward or shrug up toward your ears during each rep.

5. Resistance band row

Another fantastic lat-focused activity, this exercise also helps promote superb posture.

Try it:

Sit with your legs out in front of you (like a rowing stance) (like a rowing position).
Put the resistance band around your feet and hold both ends.
Engage your shoulder blades by pressing them together, then bring your elbows back until your hands are near your body.
Gently return to the beginning position and repeat.
Try 10–14 repetitions.

Tip: Sit up tall and straight by using your abs.

6. Standing incline chest press

Utilizing an anchor point may be very helpful, but it's not always viable, particularly if you're working out on holiday or your basement doesn't have any excellent possibilities.

This easily inclined chest press doesn't require an anchor point, so it's excellent for a home training regimen.

Try it:

Put the middle of the band beneath your left heel.
Step right foot forward so your legs are offset, with the band beneath your back foot. Holding one end of the band in each hand, position your hands at your shoulders.

Press forward and up at a 45-degree angle. Gently return to the beginning position and repeat.
Try 8–12 repetitions.

Tip: If the band is pressing against your shoulders or arms too much, change the angle of your press slightly higher, or try bending your body forward just a little further.

7. Wide-stance low crossover

Experience the strain on your inner chest muscles with this targeted low crossover.

Try it:

Put the band beneath both feet and spread your legs out wide, gripping the grips around your hips. (The broader you go, the harder you'll work your chest.)

Maintaining a small bend in your elbow, pull one handle up and in front of you, across your body, to around chest height.
Repeat on the opposite side, then continue alternating sides.
Try 8–12 repetitions.

Tips:

Keep your abs engaged.
Stop for a second at the peak of the movement to fully feel the burn.

8. High stand crossover

This is exactly like a real-deal crossover machine at the gym, but all you'll need is your handy resistance band.

This is comparable to a low crossover, except you'll anchor the band higher.

Try it:

Stand with your feet hip-width apart.

Put the resistance band at around shoulder height or a little higher on a pole (or you may use a door anchor) (or you can use a door anchor).

Facing away from the anchor point, draw the handles down and toward one another, preserving a small bend in elbows.

Hold at the bottom for a number of seconds, then gently release.

Try 8–14 reps.

Tip: You may cross your arms towards the end of the range to work your chest even more.

9. Resistance band pullover

Pullovers don't only target your pecs — that massive extension also impacts your lats and triceps as you travel through the exercise.

This works well with a flat resistance band. Handles would simply be in the way with this one.

Try it:

Attach your resistance band to a secure position low to the floor. A solid table may work if you're attempting this at home.
Lay on the floor with arms stretched above your head, gripping the band with both hands.
Keeping those arms straight, put your hands in front of your head to line up with your chest.
Hold for a few seconds before returning to the starting position.
Try 8–10 repetitions.

Tips:

Be sure to give your pecs a thorough squeeze so your chest receives the full impact of the workout.
Hold your hands close together for optimum advantage.

How to figure it out

Now, it's time to put these fantastic movements into a comprehensive resistance band chest training regimen.

It's extremely simple: Simply choose your favorite three exercises and you'll be on your way to a thorough chest workout with no weights in sight.

If you're just beginning out, consider fewer repetitions and sets. Developing strength might take time, but you've got this.

Ensure to incorporate a warmup and cooldown to prevent any undesired aches or strains.

Chapter 4

Resistance band workouts for back

It's not unusual for a training regimen to include a specific "arm day" or "leg day," so why do we shortchange the back?

A strong back is vital to sports performance and excellent posture, not to mention daily tasks – just try to operate with one that's sore or damaged. And nothing demonstrates your devotion to fitness like a pair of sculpted traps.

Yet owing to the limits of an "out of sight, out of mind" attitude, so many of us disregard our back muscles to concentrate on the ones we can readily see in the mirror.

Whether or not you ever take the time to turn around and gaze over your shoulder, your back is there... and it requires your attention!

To acquire a stronger, shapelier back, you need to push it with a range of motions.

Thankfully, you can design a dynamic exercise around just one affordable piece of equipment: the resistance band.

These are eight of the greatest resistance band back workouts.

1. Straight-Arm Lat Pull-Down

Attach a resistance band with handles to a sturdy, stationary object slightly above head height. (A door works great if you have a door anchor for the resistance band.)
Hold the grips with your arms stretched straight out in front of you and your palms facing down. Step back until you feel strain in the band. This is the starting position.
Keeping your chest up, shoulders down, and arms straight, simultaneously draw both

handles down to your sides. Pause, and then return to the starting point.

2. Band Pull-Aparts

Hold the ends of a big resistance band with both hands, palms facing down. (If your band includes handles, hold the real band below the handles to produce extra stress.)
Standing with your feet slightly apart, straighten your arms and bring them up in front of you to shoulder height. This is the starting position.
Engage your core, open your arms to your sides, and press your shoulder blades together to pull apart the band.
Gently return your arms back to the beginning position.

3. Reverse Flies

Fasten the center of a resistance band with handles to an immovable object that's around chest height.

Hold the grips of the band and, retaining a small bend in your elbows, stretch your arms straight out in front of you with your palms facing each other. Step back until you feel strain in the band. This is the starting position.

Engage your core and press your shoulder blades together as you open your arms to your sides.

Gently return your arms back to the beginning position.

4. Sitting Rows

Sit on the floor with your legs together and stretched straight in front of you. Wrap the center of a resistance band with handles over the soles of both feet, then wrap the ends of the band around the middle of each foot to produce extra resistance.

Sit up straight, engage your core, and, with the palms facing toward each other, bring both hands into your rib cage while you push your shoulder blades together.
Release your arms, allowing your hands to return to the beginning position.

5. Resistance Rows

Stand with your feet hip-width apart in the middle of a resistance band with grips. Put one end of the band around the middle of each foot and grab the handles so that your hands are facing in toward each other.
Bend your knees slightly and lean forward at the hips around 45 degrees, maintaining your back straight.
Maintain your core engaged and your back straight as you draw your hands up to your rib cage, pressing your shoulder blades together at the top.
Release your arms and repeat.

6. Superman Lat Pull

With the ends of a light resistance band in each hand, lay on your stomach with your arms stretched above, chest and arms elevated off the floor, and palms facing down. This is your starting position.
With both arms straight, draw a half-circle with your right arm, stretching it directly out to the side and down toward your right leg. Your left arm should stay straight above. Reverse the motion, gently returning to the starting position.
Repeat with your left arm, and perform equal repetitions on both sides.

7. Bird Dog Press

Stand with your feet hip-width apart in the middle of a resistance band with grips. Wrap one end of the band around the middle of each foot.

With a handle in each hand, come to your hands and knees with your hands immediately below your shoulders and your knees squarely under your hips.
Extend your banded arm in front of you and your banded leg behind you, keeping your core braced and back flat. Pause, then return to the starting point.

Do all repetitions on one side, swap arms and legs, and repeat.

Incorporate these resistance band back exercises into your regular routines or perform them back to back (ha!) for an effective workout you can do just about anywhere.

Chapter 5

Resistance band workouts for arms

Resistance band workouts for arms may be wonderful for not just developing strength, but also boosting mobility and flexibility in the upper body. Here, motions like the resistance band pull-apart, overhead resistance band stretch, and resistance band push-out may help loosen up your shoulders or alleviate stress after a long day at a desk job.

You'll need at least one band to perform the resistance band workouts for the arms below. Depending on your strength level for specific activities, you may require more than one resistance band at varying tensions so you can adapt properly.

Keep in mind that the first time around, you may need to play about to get the tension level just right. You should feel free to conduct a few practice repetitions to make sure the tension is adequately demanding. You may also use very minimal resistance and execute the techniques below as stretches, rather than as strength-building workouts.

During this workout, if you're doing 10 repetitions of an exercise, the final two reps should feel challenging, and if you had to do two to three more reps, your form would slip. If the tension seems too easy no matter how tight you pull a band, it's time to step up to a stronger band.

The Workout

1. Sitting Resistance Band Biceps Curl

Sit on a chair, bench, or stool with your feet spread.

Put one end of the resistance band beneath your left foot and grip the other end in your right hand, while resting your right elbow on your right thigh.

You may need to lean forward slightly to obtain this starting posture. I suggest keeping your core engaged and your back straight. Your left hand (that you are not using), either rest at your side or be put softly on your left thigh (as indicated) (as shown).

You should be able to start with your arm at roughly a 90-degree angle or more, with the band already tight.

Now execute a bicep curl by pushing your right hand toward your right shoulder. Keep your shoulder relaxed and concentrate on merely using your bicep to bring your hand toward you.

Perform 10-12 repetitions, then repeat on the opposite side.

Works: biceps and triceps

2. Resistant Band Rip Apart

Stand with your feet hip-width apart and grip one end of your resistance band in each hand.

Raise your straight arms to chest height, palms down, with your hands approximately 6 inches apart. The band should have a tiny degree of strain, but not be tight.

Now pull the band apart, spreading your arms wide to either side, maintaining them at the same height.

Return your arms to the center.

Works: shoulders, chest, back

3. Overhead Resistance Band Stretch

Stand with your feet together, core engaged, and grab one end of the resistance band in each hand.

With straight arms, raise the band above and maintain your hands approximately 6 inches apart so the band has some tension and is not slack.

Pull your arms apart, sweeping them down to either side, so they come to be level with your shoulders. Let the band slide behind your head (so it comes to touch your upper back) (so it comes to touch your upper back).

Return to the beginning position of holding the band above to finish the rep.

Works: triceps, back

4. Resistance Band Push-Out

Stand with your feet together, core engaged, and grasp one end of the resistance band in each hand with the band stretched across your back. Bend at your elbows to establish a 90-degree angle and let the band stretch over the midline of your back (approximately even with your sports bra strap) (about even with your sports bra strap).

At this posture, engage your back muscles by keeping your shoulders squeezed down and compress your shoulder blades as you push your arms out from your sides until your arms are completely extended.

Return to your starting posture with arms bent to 90 degrees.

Works: biceps, shoulders, back

5. Resistance Band Back Press

You may begin this move in the same location as the prior move. Stand with your feet together, core engaged, grip one end of the resistance band in each hand and wrap the band over your back.

Now take a step forward with your left foot so you are in a staggered posture. You may find this posture simpler if you expand your stance.

With your hands held at your ribcage, and the band stretched across the midline of your back, push both hands forward, completely extending your arms to chest height.

You should be utilizing your back as resistance, so remain upright, and fight the impulse to tilt forward as the band strains against your back.

Bring your arms back to your ribcage to finish the rep.

Works: biceps, chest

6. Cuff Pivot

Stand with your feet together, core engaged, and grip one end of the resistance band in each hand. You'll likely need to wrap the band a few times to get it short enough for this motion (so the tension is just perfect) (so the tension is just right).

Hold the ends of the resistance band directly below your chest (approximately even with the bottom of your ribcage), with your elbows bent and pointed out.

Holding your left hand completely stationary, draw your right hand out and toward the right, allowing the rotation to originate from your shoulder, and your elbow to naturally rotate in toward your waist. Keep a bent arm and concentrate on feeling your shoulder blades accomplish the rotational effort. Avoid the impulse to move your left arm so you're still activating muscles on both sides of your body!

Return to your starting position. Complete all of your repetitions on one side, then repeat on the other side.

Works: shoulders, rotator cuffs

7. Bow and Arrow

Stand with your feet hip-width apart and your core engaged. Hold one end of the band in each hand.

Lift both hands to chest height and stretch your left arm to your left side, maintaining your right-hand level with your sternum (Do not allow your right-hand crosses the midline of your body) (Do not let your right hand cross the midline of your body). This is your beginning position, so you may need to tweak the tension so there's little stress here, but not too much.

Now pull your right hand to the right (away from your left arm), as if bringing back an arrow in a bow. Keep your elbow pointing out and high.

Return to the starting position. Complete all of your repetitions on one side, then repeat on the other side.

Works: shoulders, triceps, chest

8. Staggered Stance Resistance Band Row

Stand with your left foot ahead of your right, so you are in a staggered posture. Widen your stance to make this posture seem simpler.

Hook the resistance band under your left foot, and grab one end of the resistance band in each hand.

Bend your left knee slightly and tilt forward at the hip so your core is engaged and your back is straight. With your arms completely stretched down toward your left foot, the band should have mild strain. That's your starting position.

Do a row pushing your hands toward your chest, and maintaining your elbows, forearms, and hands in line with your ribs.

Extend your arms to return to your starting position to finish the rep. Perform all of your repetitions on one side, then swap so the other foot is staggered ahead.

Works: triceps, shoulders

9. Resistance Band Tricep Kickback

Begin in a similar position as the preceding motion. Step your left foot forward, wrap the resistance band under your left foot, and grab one end of the band in each hand.

Bend your left knee and tilt forward at the hip, maintaining your core engaged and your back straight. Bend your elbows to 90 degrees, holding your arms tight to your sides.

From here, execute a triceps kickback by extending your arms from the elbows alone, and concentrate on maintaining the rest of your arms motionless as you press your shoulder blades together.

Re-bend your elbows to return to your starting posture. Perform all the repetitions on one side, then repeat with the other foot forward.

Works: triceps, shoulders, back

10. Tricep Reach

Stand with your feet together, core engaged, grasp one end of the band in your left hand, and hold your left hand at the small of your back so your elbow is bent.

Reach behind you to grip the opposite end of the band with your right hand and hold your right hand at shoulder height in the center (even with your spine and squarely above your left hand) (even with your spine and directly above your left hand).

From here, raise your right arm straight up over your head, stretching the band and utilizing your triceps to finish the action. Re-bend your right arm and return to shoulder height with your hand coming behind your head.

Complete all of the repetitions on one side, then repeat on the other.

Works: triceps

11. Single-Arm Front Raise

Stand with your feet hip-width apart. Wrap the band under one (or both) feet and hold one end of the band in your right hand with your right palm resting at your side. There should be little tension in the band at this initial position.

Keeping your back straight, shoulders down, and core engaged, raise your right hand straight in front of you, bringing your arm to chest height. Concentrate on utilizing your arm and shoulders alone—don't tilt your body or squeeze your shoulder to make the maneuver happen.

Lower your arm to return to your starting position. Complete all of the repetitions on one side, then repeat on the other side.

Works: shoulders

12. Single-Arm Lateral Lift With Static Hold

Stand with your feet together and loop the band under both feet, holding each end of the band in each hand.

Lift both arms to chest height, straight in front of you, with your core engaged.

Keep your left arm steady, as your swing your right arm out and to the right. Next, drop your right arm to your right side. Then reverse the action to return to your starting position.

Now keep the right arm motionless, and repeat the exercise with your left arm.

Consider the movement in two different parts: over, then down. Regulate the movement throughout: Avoid the desire to arch your arm and then let it drop to your side.

To make this action tougher, rather than rotating sides, you may keep one side steady while you execute all repetitions on a single side.

Chapter 6

Resistance band workouts for shoulders

These exercises can assist increase shoulder mobility and engage certain muscles that are crucial for stability, such as those in the rotator cuff.

1. Reverse fly

This workout strengthens your shoulders, upper back, and upper arms. It helps improve posture and is excellent for persons who sit or conduct forward-bending motions regularly.

Stand in the center of the band.
Attach the ends to opposing hands, so the band crosses in front of your lower legs.
Hinge at your hips as you bend forward slightly, maintaining your spine long and

neutral, and maintain a tiny bend in your knees throughout the action.
Drag the band upward and out to the sides until your hands are at chest height or higher.
Pull your shoulder blades together.
Maintain this posture for a few seconds.
Gently return to the starting position.

2. Front rise

This exercise strengthens your anterior (front) shoulders. To encourage appropriate posture, bring your shoulder blades down, extend your spine, and activate your abdominals.

Stand in the center of the band and grasp each end in the opposite hand, so the band crosses in front of your lower legs.
Put your palms on your thighs.
Lift your arms straight up in front of you, pausing when they're at shoulder height. Try

to prevent swinging or swaying backward as you elevate them.
Pause before gently returning to the starting position.

3. Lateral raise

This workout emphasizes your shoulders, upper back, and core muscles.

Stand in the center of the band.
Hold each end of the band in the opposite hand with your palms facing inward and the band crossed in front of your lower thighs.
Keep a small bend in your elbows as you lift your arms to the sides.
Pause for a few seconds with your arms slightly higher than your shoulder height.
Gently return to the starting position.

4. Standing row

This workout stimulates your lats and rhomboids, as well as your middle and lower trapezius. Pull your shoulder blades together as you finish the exercise. Avoid hunching your shoulders and maintain your neck flexible.

Anchor the resistance band around a doorknob or secure item.
Hold a handle in each hand, maintaining your forearms parallel to the floor.
Bend your elbows to bring your arms straight back to the sides of your ribcage.
Take caution not to arch your back or shove your ribs forward.
Gently return to the starting position.

5. Band pull-apart

This exercise strengthens your rear shoulders and upper back, helping to straighten and prevent rounded shoulders.

It also increases shoulder stability, which helps you do overhead exercises.

This exercise is good for persons who conduct tasks that force them to hunch forward. Putting your hands closer together on the band will increase the resistance.

Hold the band and stretch your arms straight out in front of you.
Lengthen your spine and keep your elbows slightly bent.
Drag the band apart as far as you can.
Pull your shoulder blades together.
Maintain this posture for a few seconds.
Gently return to the starting position.

6. Overhead band pull-apart

This workout focuses on your shoulders, back, and triceps. It enhances stability, movement, and posture.

Hold the band straight over your head.
Pull the band apart as your drop your arms to shoulder height, forcing your hands out to the sides.
Maintain this posture for a few seconds.
Gently return to the beginning position, striving to keep your shoulder blades down, away from your ears.

Have fun adding them to your exercise program, and seek the assistance of a physical therapist, doctor, or personal trainer if you'd want help or have any medical issues.

Discontinue your practice if you encounter any pain or discomfort, particularly if you're mending from an injury.

Chapter 7

Resistance band workouts for legs

Pumping iron isn't the only technique to strengthen your legs. Weight training often targets the big guns—the quadriceps, hamstrings, and glutei maximi—and neglects the smaller muscles necessary for balance and joint stability, such as the hip abductors and adductors, the flexors, and the obliques. Resistance band exercises are one of the finest methods to train every muscle in the lower body, and you can do it anywhere.

1. Fire Hydrant

The gluteus maximus—the biggest muscle in your glutes—gets the most attention when it comes to butt workouts, but practicing more movements that require abduction—moving your legs away from the midline—can help you target the smaller muscles. This fire hydrant workout works the gluteus medius and minimus by moving against the resistance of the band.

How to perform fire hydrants:

Put a resistance band slightly over your knee and get into tabletop posture with your hips precisely over your knees and your shoulders over your wrists. Using your glutes and outer thighs, pull your left leg out to the side without changing your hips. Make careful to tense your core so your upper body remains solid. Bring your left knee back to the beginning position. Continue for 10 repetitions before switching sides.

2. Tabletop Glute Kickbacks

This variant of kickbacks burns up your glutes while strengthening your core. The goal here will be to maintain your upper body and hips square and solid. A helpful visualization is to envision pushing the wall behind you with your heel. You can definitely feel your glutes working. Although this exercise mostly strengthens your lower body, it's vital to push your hands down on the ground to hold your shoulders in place.

How to execute tabletop glute kickbacks:

Put a resistance band over the arches of your feet and get into tabletop posture with your hips precisely over your knees and shoulders over your wrists. Squeezing your glutes and core, kick your left foot squarely behind you, producing a straight line from your heel to the top of your head. Continue for 10 repetitions before switching sides.

3. Glute Bridge Pulses

Glute bridges are a wonderful approach to strengthening the pelvic floor and opening up the hips. When you set a resistance band right above your knees, as demonstrated below, you're also exercising your outer thigh muscles to force your knees out. But be cautious not to elevate your hips too high to risk overriding the low back.

How to execute glute bridge pulses:

Put a resistance band on your thighs, right above your knees. Lay face up on a yoga mat with your knees bent, feet flat on the floor, and arms by your sides. Tightening your glutes and pelvic muscles, raising your hips up toward the ceiling, and pulse your hips up and down, never allowing your butt contact with the ground. Continue for 15 to 20 repetitions. For a more strenuous variant, make it a single-leg glute bridge by elevating one leg off the ground.

4. Glute Bridge With Alternating Leg Lift

Your lower abs and stability get tested with this glute bridge exercise. Raising one leg at a time with a resistance band around your thighs disrupts your balance and makes your glutes work harder to keep them raised off the ground.

How to execute a glute bridge with alternating leg raises:

 Put a resistance band around your thighs, right above your knees. Lay face up on a yoga mat with your knees bent and feet flat on the floor. Tightening your glutes and pelvic muscles, thrust your hips up toward the ceiling. While maintaining your hips up and forcing your knees out against the resistance of the band, kick your left foot out in front of you and put it back down to the ground. Push your right foot firmly on the ground to assist maintain your body steady. Next, kick your right foot out and put it back down to the ground, pushing your left foot firmly on the ground. Continue alternating sides for 15 to 20 repetitions.

5. Clamshell

Using your inner and outer thigh muscles, the clamshell exercise encourages you to move with control and concentrate on the appropriate form. Widen your thighs so the band stretches as high as you can before dropping your knee back down.

How to perform clamshells:

Put a resistance band around your thighs, right above your knees. Lay on your right side on a yoga mat and bow your knees. Put your head on your right hand or on your right forearm, and lay your left hand on your left hip. Pushing against the band, strain your glutes and thigh muscles to press your left leg out as wide as you can. Stop for a second at the peak and then gently bring your left thigh down to the starting position. This is one rep. Continue for 10 repetitions before swapping sides.

6. Resistance Band Squats

Now that you've mastered a bodyweight squat, you may ratchet up the intensity of this workout by introducing a resistance band. As He previously suggested, focus on forcing your knees out to prevent them from collapsing in. Remember to engage your core to keep your chest elevated as well.

How to perform squats:

Put a resistance band around your thighs, right above your knees. Stand with your feet hip-distance apart and stretch your arms out in front of you. Tightening your glutes and core, sit into a squat, pushing your butt back and down. Push against the resistance of the band to force your knees out. With your weight on your heels, firmly push them down on the ground to stand back up. This is one rep.

7. Resistance Band Leg Lifts

As we said before, hip abduction is a terrific approach to target the tiny muscles in your glutes. With these resistance band leg lifts, you're also actively pushing your thighs out to the sides. Want to be sure you're working the proper muscles? Place your hands on your hips to feel the muscles functioning.

How to perform resistance band leg lifts:

Put a resistance band around your ankles and stand with your feet hip-distance apart. Tightening your glutes and thighs and supporting your weight on the right leg, raise your left leg out to the side, tightening the band as far as you can without changing your hips. Moving with control, bring your left foot back to the starting position without allowing your foot strikes the ground. Continue for 10 repetitions before switching sides.

8. Glute Kickbacks

If you're weary of performing squats, these standing glute kickbacks are a wonderful way to heat up your posterior. Even before you kick your foot behind you, make careful to contract your glutes and push the opposing foot firmly on the ground to assist your balance.

How to execute glute kickbacks:

Put a resistance band around your ankles and stand with your feet hip-distance apart. Tightening your glutes and tucking your pelvis in, kick your left leg out behind you until the band is tight. Pause at the top before bringing your left foot back to the starting position. Continue for 10 repetitions before switching sides.

9. Lateral Band Walk

Although it may appear easy, your inner and outer thighs will feel the heat with this resistance band workout. Next, you want to step your feet out and in wide enough so that the band remains tight the whole time.

How to execute a lateral band walk:

Put a resistance band around your ankles and stand with your feet hip-distance apart with a small bend in the knees. Engaging your outer thighs and slightly hinging at the hips, step your left foot to the side so your feet are now shoulder-distance apart. Next step your right foot to the left, placing your feet hip-distance apart and maintaining the band taut. Alternate stepping your feet out and in for roughly 10 repetitions on each side.

10. Diagonal Band Walk

Increase your hip mobility by switching up the directions in your band walks. Much like the exercise above, the objective here is to maintain the band tight the whole time.

How to execute a diagonal band walk:

Put a resistance band around your ankles and stand with your feet hip-distance apart with a small bend in the knees. With a small bend at the hips, take a broad step up to the right side with your right foot while maintaining the band tight around your ankles, then take a wide step up to the left side with your left foot. Continue for a few repetitions before retracing your steps to walk yourself back to where you began.

Chapter 8

Resistance band workouts for core

When you speak about strengthening your core, you're usually thinking of your abs. For instance, you may be working on the rectus abdominus (that's the six-pack muscle).

The rectus abdominus flexes your spine, using muscular fibers that go up and down. It's the major mover while you're performing crunches.

But your abdominals also feature a deeper collection of muscles beneath the rectus, including the transverse abdominus, with muscle fibers that go side to side, giving both postural stability and rotation, and the oblique muscles, which are your go-to's for side-bending and rotation.

What are the muscles of the core?

Core musculature also encompasses your hips and lower back muscles, and keeping proper muscular balance is optimal for function and posture.

Having a strong core entails training for both strength and stability throughout the center of the body. When your posture is solid, you stand higher, and that enhances both form and function

How much resistance should you use? Since your abs are continually at work supporting your body, endurance is more vital than sheer strength. That is, you're better off utilizing minimal-or-no resistance with a lot of repetitions than you are with a lot of weight at low reps.

That said, with a little amount of increased stress, you can achieve increases in both strength and endurance a little more effectively. That's why resistance bands are such a terrific instrument.

Resistance bands give enough tension to engage your muscles harder without demanding the physical power required for hand weights or machines.

Also, with resistance bands, you receive lots of attention on stability and eccentric (muscle lengthening) contraction, providing you with improved postural balance with more balance on the complete core.

Resistance band workouts for abs

1. Banded bridge

Pushing onto the band helps to engage the hip abductors, which are crucial stabilizers of the hip joint and lower back.

Ideal for: beginners and beyond

With a small band around your thighs, lay face up on the ground, with your heels as near to the hips as comfortable, around shoulder-distance apart.
Raise your hips high, maintaining your shoulder blades on the ground, and softly keep the knees wide.
Keep a deep scoop in the belly as you roll the spine back down.
Perform 2 sets of 10 repetitions.

2. Mermaid twist

This workout works your obliques. To achieve the best effect, attempt to maintain your hips motionless while you spin from the waist up.

Ideal for: intermediate exercisers and beyond

Sit out to the side on one hip, with your knees bent next to you, mermaid style. Anchor the small band in your lower hand.
Hold the band near your chest with the upper hand, keep a long spine, and rotate the torso, stretching the band as you twist.
Make careful to maintain the effort in the stomach and not in the shoulders.
Do 2 sets of 6–8 repetitions on each side.

3. Banded dead bug

To train the core, make careful to maintain the spine in a steady, neutral posture throughout the activity, without arching the back.

Ideal for: intermediate exercisers and beyond

Wrap the tiny band around one foot and grasp it in the other hand.
Stabilize the hand and shoulder on the banded hand while extending the banded leg.
If you'd like, you may increase the intensity by extending the unbanded hand aloft.
Pull in your belly to support the spine as you lengthen and regulate your return to start.
Do 2 sets of 10 repetitions on each side.

4. Banded plank walk

To get the most out of this exercise, concentrate on bringing your leg forward utilizing your abdominals for control rather than overworking the hip flexors, which may cause your lower back arch.

Ideal for: advanced exercisers

Adopt a plank posture on your hands or elbows, with a band around your thighs, slightly above the knee.

While stabilizing the core, move your legs forward to a bear plank posture, with knees hovering just above the floor and back to a straight-legged plank.

Make remember to engage the abdominals and alternate the lead leg for symmetry.

Perform 2 sets of 8 repetitions, rotating the lead leg.

5. Mountain climbers

Be mindful not to compromise form while boosting speed.

Ideal for: advanced exercisers

Using the band around the arches of both feet, make your way to a straight-arm plank, feet hip-distance apart.

Switching legs, bring one knee nearer your elbows, stretch the small band, and work your core.
Do 2 sets of 15–20 complete repetitions.

6. Controlled rollup

In this situation, the band supports you on the upward portion of the action. It provides you with a reverse curl on your way down, strengthening your back and abs while relaxing the upward action.

Ideal for: beginners and beyond

Sit on the floor and wrap a resistance band around your feet, holding on with both hands.
Roll your spine down to a supine posture slowly, scooping your abdominals inside into your spine.
Nod your chin, and begin rolling up back to a sitting posture, with control. Hold your

arms as straight as possible so that the work doesn't go to the biceps.
Perform 1 set of 8–10 repetitions.

7. Russian twist

As noted above, your obliques will gain the most in rotation exercises if you concentrate on stabilizing the hips and rotating from the waist up. To preserve the lower back, be careful to maintain your spine long and avoid compressing the lumbar spine.

Ideal for: beginners and beyond

Sit in a V-sit posture, with knees bent and heels on the floor.
Wrap the band around your feet and grip the ends in both hands.
Stabilize your lower body while twisting the rib cage and bringing your hands from hip to hip with an enthusiastic speed. Repeat on the opposite side.

You can make this maneuver a bit tougher by floating your feet off the floor, and harder still by extending your legs.
Do 2 sets of 15 complete repetitions.

8. Banded bird dog

With this exercise, concentrate on engaging your hamstrings and shoulder muscles to move the band, keeping the core engaged. It's easy to arch your lower back, but attempt to maintain your spine long and powerful.

Ideal for: intermediate exercisers and beyond

On hands and knees, secure one end of the band around the arch of one foot and hold it in the hand on the opposing side.
Simultaneously stretch the banded arm and the banded knee.

Keep your spine stable and abdominals engaged and attempt to move fluidly.
Do 2 sets of 10 repetitions on each side.

9. Banded wood chop

Try your best to rotate from the torso first before tugging the band with your hands.

Ideal for: intermediate exercisers and beyond

Stand in a split stance, with the front foot anchoring one end of the band.
Both hands clasp the opposite end of the band.
Spin in the direction of the rear leg, elevating the arms to stretch the band while you maintain your core strong and hips steady.
Do 2 sets of 10 repetitions on each side.

10. Palov press

The Palov press trains your abdominals in their duty as stabilizers. Thus in this scenario, you're attempting to prevent shifting your torso while the resistance pulls on your body.

Ideal for: intermediate exercisers and beyond

Anchor the band at shoulder height and turn 90 degrees to the side.
Stretch your arms and move away from the anchor, until you feel a suitable level of strain, and then bring the elbows back in toward your chest.
Gently extend your elbows, keeping tension in the band throughout the exercise.
Try not to spin as you push the arms out in front of you. Bend your elbows to return to the starting position.
Perform 2 sets of 10 repetitions. Make careful to do both sides.

11. Double leg stretch

Try to keep your bottom rib linked to the floor and maintain a neutral spine throughout the exercise.

Ideal for: advanced exercisers

Lay on your back with your legs in a tabletop posture, bent at 90 degrees at both the hip and knee, with your feet off the ground.
Put the center of the band around your feet, and anchor the ends in your hands.
While bringing your abs down toward the floor, stretch both legs out away from your torso, and control their return. To make this exercise more demanding, you may stretch your arms above and raise your head and shoulders off the floor.
Complete 1 set of 12–15 repetitions.

Safety considerations for resistance band exercises for abs

It's vital to check for minor rips in the band before every exercise. Since elastic may snap, you want to avoid being popped in the face with a broken band. If you detect minor rips and nicks in your band, don't take a risk - replace it.

The form is particularly crucial when dealing with rising resistance.

During the muscular contraction (concentric) phase, you're likely to move in a more controlled fashion, but it's simple to forget that control during the muscle lengthening (eccentric) phase. Doing so, however, may harm both muscle and connective tissue

Maintaining a delayed release of tension may both build strength and limit the chance of injury.

Note

Resistance bands are essential equipment for exercises that you can perform anytime, anyplace.

They're portable and effective, they can provide enough resistance to build strength and endurance, and they provide enough diversity to make the exercises entertaining. Developing your core strength and posture was never so simple.

Conclusion

Utilizing resistance bands may be better than weight training in the sense that you are more in control of the tension. "You decide how far you lean into the workout, and how much your muscles are taxed as you progress into your maximum range of motion. The more power you use, the more the band will stretch, so it's like adding extra weights but without the inconvenience of moving about with parts of the apparatus.

Bands are also substantially cheaper than weights and are a fantastic alternative for novices and people resuming exercise after a hiatus. They are also incredibly lightweight and portable, so you may carry them with you when you travel on vacation or business trips.